Mogens Schou

Lithium Treatment
of Mood Disorders

A Practical Guide

6th, revised edition
1 figure and 3 tables, 2004

 Basel · Freiburg · Paris · London · New York ·
Bangalore · Bangkok · Singapore · Tokyo · Sydney

Mogens Schou

MD, Dr. med. sci., Dr. honoris causa Aix-Marseille, München, Praha, FRC Psych. (Hon.), Recipient of the Lasker Award, p.p., is Emeritus Professor of Biological Psychiatry at Århus University, Denmark. Address: Syrenvej 4, 8240 Risskov, Denmark.

1st edition 1980
2nd, revised edition 1983
3rd edition 1986
4th, revised edition 1989
5th, revised edition 1993
6th, revised edition 2004

Editions 1–5 were published under the title
Lithium Treatment of Manic-Depressive Illness

Library of Congress Cataloging-in-Publication Data
A catalog record for this title is available from the Library of Congress.

Drug Dosage

The authors and the publisher have exerted every effort to ensure that drug selection and dosage set forth in this text are in accord with current recommendations and practice at the time of publication. However, in view of ongoing research, changes in government regulations, and the constant flow of information relating to drug therapy and drug reactions, the reader is urged to check the package insert for each drug for any change in indications and dosage and for added warnings and precautions. This is particularly important when the recommended agent is a new and/or infrequently employed drug.

© Copyright 2004 by S. Karger AG, P.O. Box, CH–4009 Basel (Switzerland)
www.karger.com
Printed in Switzerland on acid-free paper by Reinhardt Druck, Basel
ISBN 3–8055–7764–8

Contents

Acknowledgments

I wish to thank the patients, relatives, nurses, general practitioners, and psychiatrists who took the time to read and comment on my manuscript.

I owe particular thanks to Paul Grof, Marylou Selo and David Chowes who gave wonderfully constructive criticism.

Mogens Schou

Foreword by a Psychiatrist

When used correctly, lithium unquestionably produces the most dramatic benefits of any medication used in psychiatry. It is clearly the treatment of choice for many who suffer from bipolar illness, effectively preventing both the manic and the depressed phases of the disorder. The primary aim of this book is to provide patients and their families with up-to-date information about the correct use of lithium – essential knowledge they will require.

When treated with lithium properly, most patients experience nothing unpleasant, but lithium has a potential to induce adverse effects. Thus, a patient who takes lithium without adequate instruction can run into trouble, just as a physician who is not well trained in its use.

Shortly after embarking on lithium prophylaxis over 40 years ago, professor Schou started writing instruction lists for his patients. Thus, this book grew out of enormous experience and out of the conviction that a well-informed patient is a critical element in effective and safe lithium treatment. It also grew out of a marked need to provide a more detailed and comprehensive instruction tool. But the book also expresses the author's intense compassion and deep respect for those suffering from manic-depressive illness and his profound understanding of their predicament.

Needless to say, professor Schou is extraordinarily well equipped for his task. Emeritus Professor of Psychiatry at the University of Aarhus and former Director of the Biological Psychiatry Laboratory at the Institute of Psychiatry at Risskov, he has pioneered the systematic use of lithium treatment in mood disorders. When he embarked on this work, psychiatric treatment was literally helpless against the capricious recurrences of manic-depressive illness. Demonstrating lithium's antimanic effect in the first double-blind trial ever carried out in psychopharmacology and subsequently proving lithium's prophylactic effect, professor Schou made a crucial contribution to a new era that has since followed. Today, when every paper on bipolar illness opens up stating that it is a recurrent illness and requires long-term treatment, it is hard to believe that prior to professor Schou's studies, there was no lasting management of the illness. But what was up to that point considered impossible suddenly became attainable: with a relatively simple element to stop the recurrences of a devastating process – manic-depressive illness.

Professor Schou not only discovered the prophylactic effect of lithium but has also remained the driving force behind the effective and safe use of lithium on a worldwide scale. In addition, more than any other work, his research has been responsible for starting the ongoing revolution in biological psychiatry. Reading this practical book for patients, written with the utmost modesty, one would never guess that the author has made such a tremendous contribution to psychiatry over the past 40 years. Because of his unique contribution, he not only received numerous awards and several honorary degrees, but was also nominated for a Nobel Prize.

Writing well for patients is the most challenging literary feat a physician can attempt. Only professor Schou knows how many dozens of drafts of this book have been earlier discarded in order to arrive at the present clarity, poignancy, and precision of writing. But it had to be done that way: well-informed patients and relatives are a critical ingredient of proper lithium treatment.

Because of the plethora of information about lithium spread in the literature, there is clearly a need for a book that reviews this knowledge and information for patients in a comprehensive manner. Professor Schou does an outstanding job in fulfilling this need, and the fact that this book is appearing in its sixth edition attests to it. The book can be best described as a remarkable compilation of the author's own extensive clinical and experimental studies over the past 50 years, plus distillation of over 20,000 reports in the literature, all masterfully condensed into about 80 pages.

I believe that every patient who either is or needs to be on lithium should own this guide, and it will be a valuable addition to the libraries of the families who live with manic-depressive illness. Because of its clarity, it will undoubtedly also serve as a useful source of information to physicians and to many healthcare professionals dealing with mood disorders.

Paul Grof, MD, PhD, FRCPC
Professor of Psychiatry, University of Ottawa
Director, Bipolar Disorders Research Unit,
Institute of Mental Health Research,
Ottawa, Canada

Foreword by a Lithium Patient

I met the author of this book when I was a recently diagnosed patient attending a conference on bipolar illness to educate myself. This was during the early 1980s. At that point I had been hospitalized 3 times for psychotic mania and psychotic suicidal depression. I was convinced that life as I had known it was over. A well-meaning psychiatric resident had prescribed lithium for me and had urged me to put up with the side effects. A social worker at the hospital had told me that I would never be able to work again. I had started doing volunteer work at Ronald Fieve's Lithium Clinic in New York. Dr. Fieve told me that there was no reason I could not continue working as a conference interpreter and tour guide and encouraged me to become a patient advocate. I did, but I was still convinced that bipolar illness could strike me down again at any point in time and that it was not worth my while to actively build up my life and pursue love, work, and personal interests. It was at this point that I met Mogens Schou. He had given an encouraging lecture on lithium and did not disappear at the end of his lecture to be whizzed back to the airport in a limousine as most other speakers. He mingled with the patients, did not sit at the VIP table reserved for lecturers at the conference, but sat among us and participated in all patient activities and self-help groups; he stated that he had come to learn from patients just as much as he had come to educate and encourage them. He told women that there was no reason not to have children because of bipolar illness or because of being on lithium. I perceived him as almost being a saint! In personal talks, he encouraged me to everything I wanted to do. I told him that if I were ever to feel better again I would go out into the world and become an inspired patient advocate. I have remained an ardent admirer of Mogens Schou, who has passionately maintained his dedication and integrity in promoting what for most of us bipolar patients is the best and cheapest medication: lithium. The reassuring part of being on lithium is that I know that it has a protective effect against suicide, and my father has committed suicide and there are quite a lot of suicides on my mother's side of the family as well.

My psychopharmacologist and I have learned to fine-tune my lithium intake so that I can live life to the fullest and regard lithium as an insurance policy, adjusting the levels to maximize the benefits and to minimize any potential side effects.

I have been a patient advocate promoting lithium for more than 20 years and I have even started a Lithium Clinic in Bolivia, where I was born and where people are so poor they cannot afford any other medication. I am convinced that Mogens Schou has returned life not only to me but to many others. I hope that with this revised book he will continue to save and restore more lives to worthwhile adventures in living!

Marylou Selo
Patient Advocate
Co-founder DBSA (Depressive and Bipolar Support Alliance, Chicago, Ill., USA – www. DBSAlliance.org), Equilibrium, Zug, Switzerland (www. Equilibrium.org)

Preface

to the 6th, Revised Edition

The first edition of this book was published in 1980 and was kindly received by readers and reviewers. Later editions have kept pace with newer developments.

Eleven years have passed since the publication of the 5th edition. Important new information can now be included. The book has been totally re-written, and a new chapter has been added about lithium's protective action against suicide.

It is the author's hope that the book will continue to be of use for patients and relatives as well as for physicians, nurses, and other care providers.

Mogens Schou

1
Introduction

Bipolar and Depressive Disorder

While the first 5 editions of this book were called *Lithium Treatment of Manic-Depressive Illness*, this edition is called *Lithium Treatment of Mood Disorders* in order to bring it in line with present-day diagnostic classification.

So what is the difference between manic-depressive illness and mood disorder? In its classical form 'manic-depressive illness' was a diagnostic unity that included manic-depressive illness with a bipolar course with both manias and depressions and manic-depressive illness with a unipolar course with depressions only and no manias. Present-day diagnostic classification distinguishes between two separate diseases, 'bipolar disorder' (or 'manic-depressive disorder' or 'manic-depressive illness'), with manias and depressions, and 'depressive disorder' (or 'major depressive disorder'), with depressions only and no manias.

Mood disorders are recognized as episodes when the patients experience alternating periods with symptoms and intervals without symptoms. In bipolar disorder there may be episodes of mania, periods with abnormal elation and increased activity, and depression, periods with abnormal sadness and melancholy. A few patients experience only manias. Occasionally the disease shows a mixture of manic and depressive features; this is referred to as a mixed state. Patients with depressive disorder have only depressions.

Bipolar and depressive disorders may start at any time of life, usually between the ages of 15 and 70 years. In general, bipolar disorder surfaces considerably earlier than depressive disorder and recurs more frequently. If bipolar disorder presents already in childhood, the clinical picture may be quite different from the picture in adults, with anxiety, phobias, eating disorders, or severe sleep disturbances.

Almost all patients experience recurrences. In both disorders there is usually a longer interval between the first and the second episode than between the second and the third. The progressive shortening of cycles and intervals later levels off. The mean number of episodes is higher in bipolar disorder than in depressive disorder.

Mania

Prominent features of manic episodes are elation, easily aroused anger, and increased mental speed. The elation varies from unusual zest to uninhibited enthusiasm. Anger manifests itself as irritability. The patients become irritated if other people do not immediately follow their many ideas. Intellectual activities take place with lightning speed, ideas race through the mind, speech flows rapidly and almost without pause, puns alternate with caustic repartee. (Spouses enjoy the periods of elation and hyperactivity much less than the patients.)

The patients' perception of themselves is changed. They are excessively self-confident and lack self-criticism. This produces a previously unknown vigor, and when that is combined with a wealth of ideas, indefatigability, and lack of inhibitions, the consequences are often unfortunate. During manic episodes patients risk spoiling their marriage, destroying their reputation, and ruining themselves financially.

Manic patients sleep very little. They rarely feel tired and are kept awake by the rapid flow of ideas. Sexual activity may be increased and the bonds of marital fidelity loosened. The patients often neglect eating and may lose weight. The combination of hyperactivity, low food intake, and too little sleep may lead to physical exhaustion.

During mania patients often fail to realize that they are ill. On the contrary, they feel unusually fit and find it difficult to understand that their nearest and dearest are of a different opinion. The situation can become very difficult, and it may be made worse by rejection and indignation from outsiders who fail to understand that illness is involved.

Depression

Depressions are in many respects the opposite of manias. They are characterized by sadness, lack of self-confidence, and decreased energy. Sadness may vary from a slight feeling of being 'blue' to black despair. The patients frequently feel painfully that their emotions are 'dried out'; they want to cry but are unable to do so. Weighed down by feelings of guilt and self-reproaches, they may consider, attempt, or commit suicide.

Patients no longer evidence courage and self-esteem. They become resigned, lacking initiative and energy. They feel that obstacles are insurmountable, have difficulty accomplishing even minor tasks, and are not capable of making even trivial decisions. Due to the low self-esteem and feelings of inadequacy patients often fear being together with other people.

The mental acuity of depressed patients is usually low. Ideas are few, thoughts move slowly, and memory function is impaired. Patients feel tired and sluggish. On the other hand, the condition may be characterized by overwhelming anxiety; patients are then agitated and restless.

Sleep is often disturbed. Occasionally there is increased need for sleep, but more often the patients have difficulty sleeping. Some patients find it hard to fall asleep, others wake up frequently, and others again wake up with a feeling of anxiety. Variations of mood can occur frequently during the course of the day. Mood is low late at night and in the early morning, everything is black, the desire to stay in bed is overwhelming, and the first few hours of the day are difficult to get through.

Depressions are often accompanied by physical changes. Muscles feel slack, facial expression is bland, and motions are slowed down. There may be constipation, menstruation may stop, and sexual interest and activity usually decrease. Appetite is reduced, and the weight may drop. Other patients may eat compulsively and gain weight.

The Nature of the Illness

Some persons are genetically predisposed to mood disorders, and there is excellent material for discovering the bipolar genes. The Genome Project has recently been completed, and now all 30,000 human genes have been identified. Researchers in many laboratories throughout the world are working on the next step: to identify how each gene affects functioning. From a research point of view, genetics of bipolar disorders currently offers the most promising and exciting developments. The findings have been converging on several regions of the human genome. Once the genes are isolated and the functioning of each relevant gene is more fully understood we may be in a position to treat patients with greater precision – in a pinpoint fashion – without side effects.

Are Patients Suffering from Bipolar and Depressive Disorder in Fact 'Patients'?

In this book I use the term 'patients' referring to persons who suffer from mood disorders, but I do it reluctantly. The term is appropriate when used for persons who are not in a manic or depressive episode, but it is more dubious when used for persons who are in an interval or for persons who are kept episode-free because of long-term lithium treatment. Under these circumstances they are not 'ill', and they may prefer to avoid the patient label with its overtones of hospitalization and passivity. However, I have not been able to find another term that is short and appropriate both for the patients themselves and for others.

Suffering from Mood Disorder

It would be more than strange if patient and family were entirely unaffected by such uprooting, violent experiences as manias and depressions. Acts carried out during manias may have unfortunate consequences. Strained relationships whether in a marriage, at work, or among friends are difficult to repair. For patients with frequent episodes it is often difficult to find their own identity because they see themselves as different persons when they are manic, when they are depressed, and when they are in remission. Perpetual watching for signs of disease may lead to an introspection that is troublesome for the patients themselves and for the family.

A special pattern is often created around patients with frequent and severe manias and depressions; spouse, children, family, and colleagues all play a role to alleviate the consequences of the incessant mood changes. The family leads a life that is dominated by fear of catastrophe, the atmosphere becomes colored by constant watchfulness, plans can only be tentative, and activities are inhibited by always having to be subordinated to the whims of the disease. Relatives are often in need of psychological support, and it is imperative that the physician keeps them informed about what is happening, especially if the patient is hospitalized.

This somber picture should, however, not obscure the fact that bipolar disorder may also bring positive experiences. These come during the mild manias with their increased self-confidence, sensitivity, and a wonderful feeling of being at-

3
Lithium Treatment of Mood Disorders

What Is Lithium?

Lithium is a metallic element that was discovered in 1818. Because it was found in a mineral, it was called 'lithium', which is derived from the Greek word *lithos*, stone. Lithium is prevalent in nature, for example in plant and animal tissues. Some lithium is mined as the mineral spodumene in North Carolina, USA, and some is extracted from brine that is pumped up from a salt desert in the Andes Mountains in Chile. Lithium and lithium compounds have many technical uses: in the production of ceramics, glass, batteries, the production of aluminum, etc.

Only small amounts of lithium are used for medicinal purposes. As a medication, lithium is always used as one of its salts, for example lithium citrate or lithium carbonate. It is the lithium part of the salt, the lithium ion, that is effective, and in principle it does not matter which salt is used.

The History of Lithium Treatment

Lithium was introduced into medical practice in 1850 for the treatment of gout. It did not work. During the following century, a number of uses were proposed, for example as a stimulant, as a sedative, for the treatment of diabetes and infectious diseases, or as a caries-preventing additive to toothpaste. Lithium was even used in the 1880s for periodic depressions, but the effect was never convincingly proved, and the treatment went out of use. Use of lithium as a taste substitute in the low-salt diet of patients with heart and kidney diseases led to serious poisonings and left many physicians with a fear of lithium.

For the treatment of hypomania lithium is superior to other treatments. If the symptoms are unlikely to be a cause for great concern, it matters little that it takes 8–10 days for lithium to take effect. Patients tolerate the more benign lithium effect better than the effect of 'straightjacket' medications.

Lithium Treatment without the Patient's Consent

It was mentioned above that treatment of mania could be made difficult because the patient does not understand that he is ill. Lithium cannot be injected, and the patient cannot be forced to swallow the pills. I am of the opinion that it is a bad idea to put crushed lithium pills into the patient's food. The appropriate dosage level is difficult to achieve, and treating a patient without his consent is likely to cause a breach of trust.

Lithium Treatment of Depression

Lithium has a therapeutic action in depressions, but antidepressants are more efficient. When antidepressants do not suffice to reduce the depressions, the adjunctive use of lithium may be helpful.

Fig. 1. The course of the disease of patients with recurrent bipolar disorder or recurrent depressive disorder who were given lithium treatment. Each row corresponds to the course of a patient from January 1, 1960, to July 1, 1969. The dark rectangles are depressions, the vertically striped ones manias, and those with oblique lines are mixed states. A slim horizontal line represents the lithium treatment. The figure shows that lithium treatment led to a lower frequency of recurrences. Many patients did not have further episodes. Some patients had recurrences during the treatment but in most cases less often than before. A few patients suffered recurrences when, against the physicians' advice, they stopped taking lithium. From Schou M: Die Lithium-Prophylaxe bei manisch-depressiven Psychosen. Nervenarzt 1971;42:1–10.

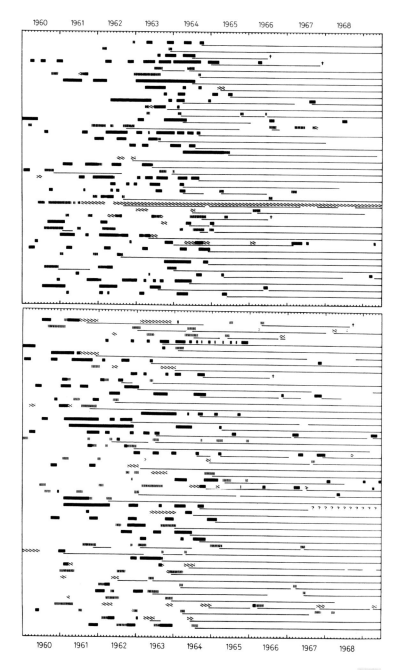

Prophylactic Lithium Treatment

Prophylaxis means prevention, but lithium cannot prevent the development of mood disorders. The term 'lithium prophylaxis' should here be understood as a procedure to prevent subsequent episodes of mania and depression. If the patients stop taking lithium, there is a risk that the disease will break out again with as frequent and severe episodes as before. Patients must therefore take lithium also during symptom-free periods.

If patients experience repeated periods of vulnerability, they can in principle be treated during these only, and long-term side effects may thereby be avoided. But in practice this procedure is time consuming and rarely used.

Prophylactic Treatment of Bipolar Disorder

Lithium was introduced in 1949 as an antimanic medication and has for many years been the 'gold standard' for prophylactic treatment in bipolar disorder.

Prophylactic Treatment of Depressive Disorder

As already mentioned, Poul Christian Baastrup and I saw in 1967 that long-term lithium treatment exerts a recurrence-preventive action not only in bipolar disorder, but also in depressive disorder. Neither then nor later did this observation have any effect on the prophylactic treatment of this disorder. The antidepressant medications had been introduced in the late 1950s, and they have later had competition only from other antidepressants and not from lithium.

It should, however, be noted that many patients are treated with antidepressants who according to present-day international classification have, or must be suspected of having, bipolar disorder. They are patients with bipolarity in the family, patients whose depressive disorder started in childhood or puberty, and patients who have had at least one episode with hypomanic symptoms. Some such patients are already treated with lithium, but many more might to their advantage be treated with lithium instead of antidepressants.

Compliance

When patients take their medicine as prescribed, they are said to be compliant, and failing compliance is the most frequent cause of recurrences during long-term lithium treatment. Lack of compliance can have many causes. The patients may have been insufficiently instructed. They can be forgetful. They may be experiencing troublesome side effects. They may stop taking lithium because it is not as effective as they had expected. Or conversely, because lithium is so effective that no further episodes develop, the patients believe they are no longer ill and therefore stop taking lithium; the outcome is usually that manias or depressions or both reappear. Some patients stop taking lithium because they dislike having their emotions controlled by medication or because they feel stigmatized for having to take psychiatric medication. They may also be under the influence of antimedication attitudes in the media or in their surroundings.

Prophylactic lithium treatment should not stand alone; it must be supported by measures to maintain compliance. Patients and their relatives must be fully informed about the nature and course of the illness and about the potential catastrophic consequences of discontinuation of treatment without the physician's consent. Patients should be advised to continue taking lithium also when they are not manic or depressed. It is the joint responsibility of patient and physician to fine-tune the medication and find the individually lowest lithium dosage and blood lithium concentration that prevent recurrences effectively. The solution to the problem of noncompliance is not to use lithium less but to use it better.

Does Lithium Gradually Lose Its Effect?

A number of medications lose their effect when they have been used for some time. Higher doses must then be given to retain the effect, or the treatment must be interrupted for a while. Lithium does not belong to that group. Even after years of use it may be fully effective, and it remains so also after stopping and later resuming treatment.

How Long Should Lithium Treatment Continue?

Lithium is taken by patients who have had repeated episodes, and to many patients it must be given for years, possibly for the rest of their lives. This does not mean that they are bound to lithium when they have once started the treatment. They can stop it at any time if it does not function satisfactorily or if significant side effects develop. Abrupt discontinuation has sometimes precipitated mania, and it is advisable to discontinue lithium gradually.

Treatment Pauses

The question has been raised whether patients in prophylactic lithium treatment may take a pause occasionally, but the risk is considerable if the patient has previously had frequent episodes.

The situation may be different for the small group of patients who have season-bound manias and depressions, for example manias and depressions that occur every winter and spring. Such patients may be tempted to stop treatment during the summer and start it again in late fall. But there are problems. The season-bound rhythm may have changed, and it can take some time before the prophylactic effect sets in again. I tend to advise against treatment pauses.

Quiet before the Storm

To be freed of depressions is a clear advantage. To no longer experience manias may be a mixed blessing as there are patients who miss the hypomanic episodes. Some patients who occasionally feel that a hypomania is in progress while the treatment is keeping the lid on have raised a question that is worth discussing: is it possible to lower the lithium dose to the point that the hypomania develops to a pleasant and constructive degree, yet does not develop into a full-blown, potentially destructive, mania?

I know that patients have done so and enjoyed it. One of them spoke enthusiastically about the 'silver lining' of hypomania. The patients may use such periods to accomplish a particular piece of work or to achieve a certain goal. In order to venture such an experiment the patients must, however, have extensive experience with their disease and with the course of an upcoming mania. Owing to flowering ideas and excess of energy, the latter is often accompanied by sleeplessness, and lack of sleep may in itself aggravate a hypomania into a full-grown mania. The quiet before the storm may develop into a destructive tornado.

When Should Lithium Not Be Given?

Lithium treatment must not be given to patients with severe kidney disease, serious heart disease, or diseases related to disturbances of fluid or salt balance, and the treatment should be interrupted during high fever. The kidney function falls with advancing age, but this does not mean that old people should not take lithium. They should be given lower doses.

How Does Lithium Work?

We do not know fully – yet. Lithium has a large number of biological effects, but it is difficult to know which effect or effects are related to the action of lithium on mood disorders, for the cause of these disorders is still unknown. Particularly important progress has shown that lithium has a protective effect on brain tissue and increases gray matter where there has previously been shrinkage due do depression. The clinical relevance of these findings is not yet clear. These and other hypotheses are being investigated, and the nut *will* be cracked.

4
Other Prophylactic Medications

There is a need for other recurrence-preventing medications in patients who do not respond fully to lithium and in patients with troublesome side effects. During the last 24 years the chase after substitutes for lithium has been intense.

Medication trials have shown that antiepileptics, medications used in the treatment of epilepsy, may be as good as lithium, and they are now used extensively. One should, however, note that investigations from recent years have shown that the efficacy of prophylactic medications depends first and foremost on the patients who are treated. In patients with *typical* bipolar disorder, those who are completely free of symptoms in the intervals and in whose family there may be bipolar disorder, lithium is clearly the best prophylactic medication. In patients with more *atypical* bipolar disorder, those who have symptoms also during the intervals and who may have other psychiatric illnesses in the family, some of the antiepileptic medications are the most effective. It can, for example, be carbamazepine (Tegretol), valproate (Deprakine), or lamotrigine (Lamictal).

5
Lithium Protection against Suicide

The most tragic outcome of mood disorder is suicide. This risk is considerable. In mood disorders the mortality due to suicides is higher than it is of most heart diseases and many types of cancer. The mortality of mood disorders is 2–3 times higher, and the suicide-related mortality is 20–30 times higher than in the general population.

In the 1980s it was noted that the frequency of suicides was conspicuously low among lithium-treated patients in three major mood disorder clinics in the USA, and systematic investigations from the 1990s indicated that long-term lithium treatment is associated with a markedly reduced frequency of suicide attempts and completed suicides. Studies in which the same patients were followed on and off lithium have been particularly impressive. The frequency of suicide attempts and of completed suicides is 10–15 times lower in patients who are on lithium than in those who are not.

It would be wrong to claim that an antisuicidal effect of lithium has been definitively proved. Such proof is in principle not possible for any kind of antisuicidal intervention for there is no matching patient group to compare with. After all, one cannot keep suicide-threatened patients on placebos or deprived of psychological and social support merely to observe if and when they will commit suicide. Nor can one determine by throwing a dice when and in whom an ongoing and possibly effective intervention should be discontinued.

But the studies reviewed are not *incompatible* with the assumption that lithium has a striking antisuicidal effect. As scientists, the psychiatrists must concede that the investigations only indicate such a possibility. As responsible clinicians, they owe it to patients and relatives alike not to disregard that possibility. It is difficult to understand why lithium is not used as an antisuicidal medication in patients with depressive disorder, in patients with bipolar disorder, and in patients with schizophrenia, who have severe depressions, thoughts about committing suicide, suicide attempts in the past, or suicides in the family.

6
Being in Lithium Treatment

Benefits from Long-Term Lithium Treatment

It was described above how affective disorders may interfere with the life and well-being of patient and family, how the attacks of the disease may lead to dysfunction and destruction, and how the intervals between attacks may become dominated by uncertainty, tension, and fear of the future.

All this is altered by successful lithium treatment. Recurrences become fewer and milder, or they may disappear completely. The patients once more become the persons they were before they became ill. Spouses describe how the patient is now 'on an even keel', 'in much better shape than he has been for years', 'able to cope with difficult situations much more adequately', 'again her own self as she was when we married', etc.

After years of living with a foreboding fear it may be difficult to hope again, but gradually patient and family experience how the course of the disorder has changed; the patient is now less fearful, ambiguous, and indecisive. Patients feel that life becomes once more safe and predictable and that normal relationships can be established or re-established. A patient wrote: 'Above all it is gratifying to be trusted, and that people around you start making normal demands on you.' For patients whose existence was dominated by frequent and severe recurrences, treatment with lithium may improve their quality of life miraculously.

Perhaps the most important difference lithium makes for patients and relatives is the knowledge that as long as the patients are in prophylactic treatment, their risk of attempting or committing suicide is 10–20 times lower than when they are not.

(This chapter has dealt with the benefits to the patients. On a more materialistic note one might ask what society gains from lithium treatment. It has been estimated that in the USA between 1970 and 1991 lithium saved society close to USD 170 billions or an average of over USD 8 billions per year.)

Problems

Lithium treatment is of unquestionable value to many patients; the patients' families and friends almost always react with an immense feeling of relief on seeing the result of successful lithium treatment. But those who are close to the patients may need time to adjust to the new situation. This is best illustrated by the effect of lithium treatment on marital relations. In most cases the marital climate is markedly improved during lithium treatment, but occasionally the spouse misses the enthusiasm and sexual intensity the patient showed during mild manias.

Successful lithium prophylaxis may also lead to a radical reshuffling of roles and responsibilities in the family. The main repercussions can affect the spouse, whose central role as upholder of home and family is endangered by the patient's recovery and who may therefore sabotage the treatment covertly or openly. Spouse, patient, and physician must work together on these problems.

Cooperation between Patient and Therapeutic Team and between Patients Themselves

Prophylactic lithium treatment places a responsibility on both patient and physician; both must cooperate in order to achieve the best possible results. Persons in lithium treatment are not 'ill', and they should try to replace the passive patient role with an active effort.

The physician's interest must include the patients' general welfare and experiences during the treatment, positive as well as negative ones, and if problems arise, they must be taken up for discussion. It is important for the patients to know that the physician is available and has time.

If patients have attended a mood disorder outpatient clinic for some time and then, as is frequent in Denmark and some other countries, are transferred to their general practitioners' care, they should continue to come to the clinic at intervals agreed upon between patient and psychiatrist. The patients come for blood tests and for a talk with the psychiatrist. It is the patients' and the family's responsibility that the patient shows up for these appointments, and if they do not, it may be the secretary's responsibility to contact and remind them. Without a lifelong follow-up the patients tend to drop out of the treatment, and then the disorder may return.

In many countries there are patient-run support groups, also called self-help groups, where newcomers meet experienced peers in order to share experiences, learn from each other, and discuss problems (for a list of support groups in various countries, see page 69).

7
Practical Management of the Treatment

Preparations

Table 1 shows preparations marketed in English-speaking countries. I have tried to provide as exact information as possible, but I cannot be held responsible for errors in or omissions from the table.

Most of the pills contain lithium carbonate, the remaining 3 contain lithium citrate, but this does not matter because it is the lithium ion that is active. It is more important that different preparations have different lithium contents. Change from one preparation to another may therefore require that a different number of pills must be taken. The lithium dose, expressed in millimoles (mmol), should remain the same.

It does not matter whether lithium is taken with a meal, but the pills should be washed down with ample amounts of water. Another possibility is to take the pills in yoghurt. It is not essential that the pills be taken at exactly the same time every day, but on the day before the visit to the laboratory the last dose must be taken 12 h (11–13 h) before the blood sample is drawn. Lithium pills are best stored in a dry place and out of reach of children. Some of the pills are of the so-called slow-release type. They release lithium more slowly in the intestines and should be swallowed, not crushed or chewed.

Some patients find it difficult to remember to take their pills, at least until they have established a treatment routine. We are dealing with prophylactic treatment, and much of the time there are no symptoms to remind the patients of the pills. It may be an advantage to use clear plastic containers with a separate compartment for each day of the week. If the container is filled up on a particular weekday, there is not much to remember during the week, and it can be seen at a glance whether any pills have been forgotten. If this has happened, the patient should not try to make up by taking more pills the next time. One or 2 omissions usually do not matter much.

Table 1. Lithium preparations marketed in English-speaking countries

Name	Drug company	Lithium salt	Amount of salt mg	Amount of lithium mmol	Type
Camcolit-400	Norgine, UK	carbonate	400	10.8	slow release
Carbolith	ICN, Canada	carbonate	300	8.1	conventional
Cibalith-S	Ciba-Geigy, USA	citrate	752 in 5 ml	8.0 in 5 ml	syrup
Duralith	Janssen	carbonate	300	8.1	slow release
Eskalith	Smith Kline Beecham, USA	carbonate	300	8.1	conventional
Eskalith CR	Smith Kline Beecham, USA	carbonate	300	8.1	slow release
Liskonum	Smith Kline Beecham, UK	carbonate	450	12.2	slow release
Litarex	CD, UK	citrate	564	6.0	slow release
Lithane	Pfizer, Canada	carbonate	300	8.1	conventional
Lithicarb	Protea, Australia	carbonate	250	6.8	conventional
Lithium Phasal	Pharmax, UK	carbonate	300	8.1	slow release
Lithobid	Ciba-Geigy, USA	carbonate	300	8.1	slow release
Lithonate	Solvay Pharmaceuticals, USA	carbonate	300	8.1	conventional
Lithotabs	Solvay Pharmaceuticals, USA	carbonate	300	8.1	conventional
Manialith	Muir & Neil, Australia	carbonate	250	6.8	conventional
Priadel	Delandale, UK, and Protea, Australia	carbonate	400	10.8	slow release
Priadel Liquid	Delandale, UK	citrate	520 in 5 ml	5.5 in 5 ml	syrup

Type of Pills and Number of Daily Doses

The reason why blood samples must be drawn about 12 h after the last lithium dose is that the concentration varies during the day and night. When 1 dose is taken in 24 h, the lithium concentration rises to a maximum after 2–4 h and then drops again. If a patient takes 2 doses per day, the curve has 2 peaks. When the blood sample is drawn 12 h after taking lithium, the lithium concentration varies least. The variation may be smaller when slow-release pills are used and when 2 doses are taken instead of 1. The most significant procedure for avoiding side effects is to use as low doses and serum lithium concentrations as are compatible with a satisfactory treatment response.

Laboratory Tests

Before lithium treatment is started, the patient is examined by a physician and asked about previous and present illnesses; in addition laboratory tests are carried out to check the physical condition. They usually include examination of blood and urine, an electrocardiogram, and assessment of blood pressure.

Lithium treatment routine includes follow-up with regular laboratory tests. The most important are determination of the lithium concentration in the blood and a creatinine test to check the kidney function. The thyroid function may be examined at longer intervals. Blood samples are drawn from a vein in the elbow. The patient needs not fast. Serum lithium is determined once a week during the first few weeks to support the dose adjustment.

Patients in lithium treatment should be able to serve as blood donors, but owing to a lack of familiarity with lithium treatment this is not considered acceptable practice in many countries.

The recommendations given here deal with minimum requirements for laboratory monitoring under ordinary circumstances, but sometimes circumstances are not ordinary. In developing countries badly needed lithium treatment may not be instituted because of the lack of laboratory facilities, and in countries without a socialized health system poor patients may be deprived of this treatment because they cannot afford regular laboratory examinations. In my opinion it is responsible practice to prescribe lithium even without laboratory monitoring and instead provide close clinical monitoring and dosage adjustment if the alternative is that no prophylactic therapy is given at all.

Dosage Adjustment in Prophylactic Lithium Treatment

The daily dosage requirement differs individually and may range from 2–3 pills to about 20–30 pills. Frequently used prophylactic doses are 2–4 pills daily.

There are two reasons why dose requirements differ. First, different patients excrete lithium with different rates so that they may need different doses to achieve the same blood lithium concentration. Secondly, the sensitivity of different people differs so that different patients must be adjusted to slightly different blood lithium levels.

Since the patients' excretion and sensitivity are not known in advance, dosage adjustment must be a stepwise procedure. One starts with 1 pill per day for a week. This dose is so small that it will be harmless and without side effects even for sensitive patients with a low excretion rate. Thereafter the lithium concentration in the blood is determined, and the dosage is adjusted to give a lithium concentration within a standard range that is 0.6 mmol/l or higher and 0.8 mmol/l or lower. A week later the lithium concentration is determined again in order to see whether it is within the standard range, and, if needed, another adjustment is made. The further frequency of concentration controls is agreed upon between patient and physician.

There are elderly patients who do not tolerate and do not need lithium levels higher than 0.3–0.4 mmol/l. Other patients can only be protected effectively against recurrence if their blood lithium concentration is between 0.8 and 1.0 mmol/l. Blood lithium concentrations lower than 0.3 mmol/l are inactive in most patients, and blood concentrations higher than 1.0 mmol/l are often accompanied by serious side effects and may involve a risk of poisoning.

It is noteworthy that in the USA the recommended lithium levels are higher than those recommended here. This is because an American study of 1989 compared doses leading to what the authors called 'standard' lithium levels, 0.8–1.0 mmol/l, with doses leading to low levels, 0.4–0.6 mmol/l. The trial suggested that the former levels might be more effective but were also associated with more side effects than the latter. The authors nevertheless chose to recommend the high levels. They did not examine effects and side effects of levels between 0.6 and 0.8 mmol/l. There are consequently more side effects when the American recommendations are followed than when the European recommendations are followed.

Also within the standard range of 0.6–0.8 mmol/l, delicate adjustment of the dosage is important. Patient and physician must together find the optimum lithium level, and even changes as small as 0.1 or 0.2 mmol/l upwards or downwards may alter the patient's quality of life. If lithium is too low, recurrences of mania and depression threaten. If lithium is just right, senses are sharper, emotions deeper, and life richer.

During the last months of pregnancy lithium is excreted more rapidly through the kidneys, and at the time of delivery the excretion falls abruptly to pre-pregnancy values. Blood lithium should therefore be tested at relatively short intervals and the dosage adjusted accordingly. It may be advisable to stop lithium treatment a few weeks before delivery and re-start it soon after.

8
Side Effects

As other active medications lithium may have side effects, and they can possibly become so severe that the patient prefers to stop the treatment. But in most cases the side effects are mild and a modest price to pay for the emotional stability achieved.

Physical Side Effects

During treatment the patients may suffer from *thirst* and *urine production exceeding the normal.* This may disturb sleep during the night and cause social embarrassment during the day. In these patients the kidneys cannot concentrate the urine to a normal extent, and the urine volume therefore increases. Increased urine production over an extended period can lead to dehydration and may in fact be so dangerous that the lithium treatment has to be stopped. The remedy is not to drink less. On the contrary, the patients should be careful to quench their thirst. The extra urine production may be counteracted by a lowering of the lithium dosage under supervision of a physician. The kidneys then regain their concentrating ability, but this can take some months.

During lithium treatment patients may *gain weight.* Weight gain is on the average 4 kg (about 10 lb), but this can vary widely. Some patients do not gain weight at all, and others gain more. Weight gain usually occurs within the first 6–12 months, and thereafter the weight stabilizes. Increase in weight is more likely if lithium is taken together with antidepressant drugs, and if the patients already weigh too much.

Prevention is the main factor in fighting weight gain. Exercise and a sensible diet can often keep the weight down. The patients should avoid drinking calorie-rich beverages. It is particularly important that thirst be quenched with water, tea or coffee without sugar, and sugar-free soft drinks. Reducing the lithium dosage may be helpful. Drastic slimming diets should be avoided.

Tremor (trembling) of the hands may be an aggravation of a family tremor or may develop independently. In most cases it is so weak that it is scarcely perceived by others, but some patients may find it troublesome in their vocation (surgeon, watchmaker, some sport players), and they may be embarrassed at parties when they have to grip the glass with both hands in order not to spill. The tremor may be aggravated when the patients are tired and tense and also after smoking and intake of coffee. Simultaneous treatment with antidepressant medication increases the tendency to develop tremor. This side effect can be counteracted by a lowering of the lithium dosage or by treatment with propranolol (Inderal). The patient may take 10–20 mg of propranolol half an hour before a party or an important meeting.

During lithium treatment the thyroid gland may increase in size *(goiter)*, or the thyroid function may decrease, resulting in lowered metabolism *(myxedema)*. The family usually discovers the neck swelling, or the patient feels that his shirt collar has become too tight. The diagnosis of myxedema can be missed because some of its symptoms resemble a slight depression with fatigue, decreased vitality, sadness, and slow reactions. Determination of the level of thyroid-stimulating hormone in the blood can clear up the diagnosis. Once goiter or myxedema has been diagnosed, it is easy to treat. Thyroid hormone (thyroxine) is taken together with lithium.

Lithium may have other side effects, but they are rare.

Risk and Risk Situations

For most patients lithium is without risk and not a capricious medication. Risk of toxicity arises in particular situations, and by avoiding these, the patients may contribute to the safety of the treatment.

Table 2 shows a list of the signs that patient and family will be wise to remember. If one or more of these signs become prominent, the physician should be informed so that he can examine the patient and check the blood lithium concentration. Patients with impending intoxication should stop the lithium intake and drink plenty of water. Lithium intoxication is treated with water and in severe cases possibly with rinsing of the blood (dialysis).

Depressed patients have occasionally tried to commit suicide by swallowing many lithium pills, usually without reaching their desperate goal. Intoxication caused by an acute overdose seems to be less dangerous, although hardly less unpleasant, than a gradually developing lithium intoxication.

Table 2. Signs of impending lithium intoxication

Dullness	Sleepiness
Heaviness of limbs	Unsteady gait
Indistinct speech	Increased tremor
Nausea	Diarrhea

Table 3. Risk situations during lithium treatment

Dehydration	High fever
Low salt intake	Protracted vomiting and diarrhea
Rigorous dieting	Unconsciousness for several hours
Anesthesia and major operations	

Table 3 shows risk situations during lithium treatment. The patients should be particularly attentive to situations involving the risk of dehydration and should consume ample amounts of fluid. They must not neglect feelings of thirst for any prolonged time, and they are advised to bring extra fluid when it is difficult to have something to drink, for example on long car trips or walking tours. Salt intake is also important.

Lithium treatment should be stopped before a (nonacute) operation with full anesthesia and not be resumed until fluid and salt balance are restored. Tell your physicians that.

Interaction

Two medications given together may result in interaction, that is mutual strengthening or weakening of each other's effects. Both patient and physician must remember the possibility of interaction.

Diuretics are usually safe medications, but taken with lithium they may not be. They promote the excretion of water and may lead to dehydration with a risk of intoxication.

Other medications against *increased blood pressure* such as for example verapamil should be avoided.

Many medications used against *rheumatism* interact with lithium and should be avoided. Medications as for example acetylsalicylic acid (Aspirin) and indomethacin (Indocid) should, however, be safe, but it is important that the lithium concentration is checked regularly:

The effects of *herbs and other medicinal plants* on the body are not known, and it is best not to take them.

Drinking coffee has no effect if the same amount is consumed every day, but if the patient changes from drinking much coffee to drinking little, it may be necessary to lower the lithium dosage.

Lithium may lower the sensitivity to alcohol, and it is best to limit the alcohol intake to 1–2 glasses.

There should be no interaction between lithium and other medications, but one must always remember that side effects may have been caused by interaction.

There is no interaction between lithium and birth control pills.

Cognitive and Emotional Side Effects

The quality, kind, and frequency of side effects to the mind are subject to discussion because affective illness itself may influence not only mood but also the ability to remember and reason, and it can be difficult to distinguish between what is caused by lithium and what by the illness.

Most patients in lithium treatment feel normal and function normally. But some, especially those who are usually hypomanic, feel that lithium treatment has changed their personality. Life is grayer than before; there is less enthusiasm, energy, and determination. Reactions are not as quick as they used to be, nor memory as astute. A patient regretted that in discussions he was no longer able to obtain the level of excitement he considered necessary, commenting 'Doctor, I am a politician and *must* get excited when I discuss'. These patients may experience relief after reduction of the dosage, because they feel that their ordinary selves return.

Male patients occasionally complain of decreased potency during lithium treatment, but it is not clear whether this is a lithium effect, a sign of slight depression, or a coincidence.

Cognitive side effects are readily reversible and disappear when the lithium dose is reduced or the treatment discontinued.

Lithium and Creative Work

Patients occasionally report that lithium treatment lowers their flow of ideas, fantasy, and productivity, and that their creative ability has been weakened. These are serious disadvantages for persons whose professional work is based on the ability to translate them to practical, scientific, or artistic productivity. However, long-term lithium treatment is given to persons with frequent episodes of mania or depression or both, and these attacks may in themselves affect creative work. So the question is what to prefer, the illness or the treatment.

In order to gain an impression of advantages and disadvantages, I contacted a number of artists whose illness had been brought under control by lithium and asked them what had happened to their creative ability. Out of 24 artists, 6 felt that ideas now came less readily and that their productivity had declined during lithium treatment. Four of them stopped lithium for this reason. They preferred to maintain the inspiration and energy of the mild manias and were in return willing to risk depressions and severe manias. Two hereafter had recurrence of the illness.

Six artists reported that their productivity had remained unaltered, and there were finally 12 artists who felt that they created more during lithium treatment than before. Their depressions had been painful and artistically barren, and their manias had been dominated by valueless hyperactivity. During lithium treatment, they could function with steadiness and better artistic discipline to the advantage of both the quantity and the quality of their work.

9

Pregnancy, Delivery and Breastfeeding

Malformations

Early experiments on primitive aquatic animals had shown that exposure to high concentrations of lithium in the surrounding fluid led to malformations of the offspring. This is called a teratogenic effect. After lithium had first been used for the treatment of manic-depressive patients in 1949, a 'Register of Lithium Babies' was established in 1969 in order to give warning if malformed children should be born by mothers having been in lithium treatment during pregnancy. The register was based on voluntary reports, and it indicated an increased frequency of congenital malformations of the heart. However, these findings exaggerated the risk because congenitally malformed babies were more likely to have been reported than normal babies, and the retrospective register was closed in 1990. When the lithium baby register was started, psychiatrists were not used to think along teratogenic lines, and the register's estimate of the *maximum* teratogenic risk was taken as a measure of lithium's *true* teratogenic effect. That gave lithium a 'bad press'. Later investigations without the bias of the register have given reassuring results. Lithium can be given safely during the last 6 months of the pregnancy, and if the risk of recurrence is high, it can also be given during the first 3 months. The risk of fetal changes is minimal.

The 'Lithium Babies' at Five

Most lithium babies – children of women who had taken lithium during the pregnancy – are born without malformations, but it seemed conceivable that they might reveal developmental abnormalities later. Therefore a study was made of all Scandinavian lithium children who were born without malformations and who had reached the age of 5 years or more. Their intellectual and physical developments were compared with those of their brothers and sisters who had not been exposed to lithium in the womb. The study did not reveal any differences between the groups.

Breastfeeding during Lithium Treatment

Small amounts of lithium pass from the mother's blood to her milk and hence to the nursing child. For this reason I have in previous editions of this book advised women in lithium treatment to bottle-feed their babies. However, breastfeeding plays an important role for both mother and child, physically and psychologically, and it is today doubtful whether it is advisable to abstain from breastfeeding during lithium treatment. It is now possible to measure the lithium concentration in the mothers' milk, and it is still lower than in the blood of the fetus.

10
Epilogue

So now we come to the bottom line. I have written about something that is unpleasant, namely side effects, and something that is necessary, namely treatment management and control. The book is meant to give sober information. The many, many patients around the world who are treated successfully with lithium give strong evidence that in almost all cases the plusses outweigh the minuses.

Supplementary Reading

Alda M: Genetic factors and treatment of mood disorders. Bipolar Disord 2001;3:318–324.

Angst J, Sellaro R: Historical perspectives and natural history of bipolar disorder. Biol Psychiatry 2000;48:445–457.

Duke P, Hochman G: A Brilliant Madness: Living with Manic-Depressive Illness. New York, Bantam Books, 1992.

Goodwin FK: Rationale for long-term treatment of bipolar disorder and evidence for long-term lithium treatment. J Clin Psychiatry 2002;63(suppl 10):5–12.

Goodwin FK, Ghaemi SN: The impact of the discovery of lithium on psychiatric thought and practice in the USA and Europe. Aust NZ J Psychiatry 1999;33:S54–S64.

Goodwin FK, Jamison KR: Manic-Depressive Illness. Oxford, Oxford University Press, 1990.

Grof P: Excellent lithium responders: People whose lives have been changed by lithium prophylaxis; in Birch NJ, Gallichio VS, Becker RW (eds): Lithium: 50 Years of Psychopharmacology. New Perspectives in Biomedical and Clinical Research. Cheshire, Weidner Publishing Group, 1999.

Grof P: Selecting effective long-term treatment for bipolar patients: Monotherapy and combinations. J Clin Psychiatry 2003;64(suppl 5):53–61.

Jamison KR: Touched with Fire: Manic-Depressive Illness and the Artistic Temperament. New York, MacMillan, 1993.

Jamison KR: An Unquiet Mind: A Memoir of Moods and Madness. New York, Knopf, 1995.

Jamison KR: Night Falls Fast – Understanding Suicide. New York, Knopf, 1999.

Jefferson JW, Greist JH, Ackermann DL, Carroll JA: Lithium Encyclopedia for Clinical Practice, ed 2. Washington, American Psychiatric Press, 1987.

Johnson FN: The History of Lithium Therapy. London, MacMillan, 1984.

Müller-Oerlinghausen B, Berghöfer A, Bauer M: Bipolar disorder. Lancet 2002;359:241–247.

Müller-Oerlinghausen B, Greil W, Berghöfer A (eds): Die Lithiumtherapie: Nutzen – Risiken – Alternativen, ed 2. Berlin, Springer, 1997.

Schou M: Phases in the development of lithium treatment in psychiatry; in Samson F, Adelman G (eds): The Neurosciences: Paths of Discovery II. Boston, Birkhäuser, 1992.

Woggon B: Ich kann nicht wollen! Berichte depressiver Patienten. Bern, Huber, 1998.

Wyatt RJ, Henter ID, Jamison JC: Lithium revisited: Savings brought about by the use of lithium 1970–1991. Psychiatr Q 2001;72:149–166.

Support Alliances Dealing with Depression and Bipolar Disorder

Australia
Bipolar Disorder Meetup
Perth
Website bipolar.meetup.com/members/87

Fyreniyce (Fire and Ice)
E-Mail Fyreniyce-subscribe@egroups.com

Austria
SHG
SHG Neunkirchen
Peisinger Strasse 19
AT–2620 Neunkirchen (Austria)
E-Mail psychiatrie@khneunkirchen.at

Club D&A (Depression and Anxiety) – Clubzentrum Wien
Schottenfeldgasse 40/8
AT–1080 Wien (Austria)
Tel. +43 407 7227 71
E-Mail office@club-d-a-a.at

Belgium
VVMD (Flemish Association of Manic Depressives)
Tel. +32 53 77 50 97
E-Mail vvmd.vzw@belgacom.net

Psychoarts 2000
E-Mail luc.leysen@klina.be

Brazil
Apolar
E-Mail apolar@silvanprado.psc.br
Website www.silvanprado.psc.br

Canada
Mood Disorders Society of Canada
3–304 Stone Road West
Guelph, Ontario N1G 4W4 (Canada)
Tel. +1 519 824 5565
E-Mail washdown@shaw.ca
Website mooddisorderscanada.ca

Denmark
DepressionsForeningen
Vendersgade 22
DK–1363 Copenhagen (Denmark)
Tel. +45 3312 4727
E-Mail depression@inet.uni2.dk

France
France Dépression
Association française contre la dépression et la maladie maniaco-dépressive
Association Loi 1901
4, rue Vigée-Lebrun
FR–75015 Paris (France)
Tel. +33 1 4061 0566
E-Mail france.depression@libertysurf.fr

Germany
DGBS Deutsche Gesellschaft für Bipolare Störungen e.V.
PO Box 920249
DE–21132 Hamburg (Germany)
Tel. +49 40 85408883
E-Mail dgbs.ev@t-online.de
Website www.dgbs.de

Ireland
Mood Disorder Fellowship of Ireland
Fenian Chambers
3738 Fenian Street
Dublin 2 (Ireland)
(May no longer exist; has no website)

Italy
IDEA
Milan
(May no longer exist; has no website)

Netherlands
VMDB (Association of Manic Depressives and Care-Givers)
PO Box 24076
NL–3502 MB Utrecht (The Netherlands)
Tel. +31 30 260 3030
E-Mail mbakhuis@dds.nl
Website www.vmdg.nl

Spain
Associació de Bipolars de Catalunya (ABC)
C-Cuba, 2
Hotel d'Entitas 'Can Guardiola'
ES–0830 Barcelona (Spain)
Tel. +34 93 274 14 60 and +34 93 274 93 38
E-Mail cen00abc@jazzfree.com

Alianza para la Depresión
General Margallo 27
ES–28020 Madrid (Spain)
E-Mail smith@alianzadepresion.com

Switzerland
Equilibrium (founded in 1994)
Obernhofstrasse 8
CH–6340 Baar (Switzerland)
Tel. +41 848 143 144
Website www.depressionen.ch

United Kingdom
Manic Depressive Fellowship
Castle Works, 21 St. George's Road
London SE1 6ES (UK)
Tel. +44 207 793 2600
E-Mail mdf@mdf.org.uk

Depression Alliance
Tel. +44 845 123 2320
Website www.depressionalliance.org

Manic Depressive Fellowship Scotland
Mile End Mill – Studio 10/9
Abbey Mill Business Centre
Seed Hill Rd.
Paisley PA1 1TJ (UK)
E-Mail manic@globalnet.co.uk

USA
Child and Adolescent Bipolar Foundation
(On-line support and education for parents, teachers and kids)
PMB 331
1187 Wilmette Ave.
Wilmette, IL 60091 (USA)
Tel. +1 847 256 8525
Fax +1 847 920 9498
E-Mail cabf@bpkids.org
Website www.bpkids.org

Depression and Bipolar Support Alliance (DBSA) (founded in 1986)
(Previously National DMDA – Depressive and Manic-Depressive Association)
730 N. Franklin Street, No. 501
Chicago, IL 60610 (USA)
Tel. +1 800 626 3632
Website www.dbsalliance.org

Mood Disorders Support Group/New York (MDSG) (founded in 1986)
PO Box 30377
New York, NY 10011 (USA)
Tel. +1 212 533 6374
Website www.mdsg.org

Subject Index